Living With A Ghost

Who We Are and Why We Do What We Do

MICHAEL T. RAILEY, M.D.

Living With A Ghost

Who We Are and Why
We Do What We Do

© 2025 Michael Railey, MD
Living With A Ghost, Who We Are And Why We Do What We Do

No part of this book may be reproduced in any written, electronic, recording, or photocopying form without written permission of the publisher. The exception would be in the case of brief quotations embodied in critical articles or reviews and pages where permission is specifically granted by the publisher.

Scripture quotations are from The Holy Bible, The New Open Bible Study Edition (KJV) © 1990 by Thomas Nelson, Inc. Other Scriptural References are from Biblegateway.com.

Although every precaution has been taken to verify the accuracy of the information contained herein, the author and publisher assume no responsibility for any errors or omissions. Names have been changed for privacy purposes. No liability is assumed for damages that may result from the use of information contained within. Scriptural references are from Biblegateway.com; several versions have been used. All rights reserved worldwide.

Published in the United States, Mission Possible Press, a Division of Absolute Good Enterprises. AbsoluteGoodEnterprises.com

Author Contact: Dr. Michael Railey
raileymt@gmail.com

ISBN: 978-1-7352454-8-5

Dedication

This book is dedicated to those people like myself who refuse to live their lives tolerating their flaws and unchecked personal challenges which have been destructive to them. Emotional wounds which haunt us throughout life keep us incomplete and broken.

We instead seek help from God in choosing to look in the mirror, forgetting not what we see. We fight to gain God's best will for our lives. I can assure you that you will rejoice in your efforts as the result of your spiritual revelations toward self-improvement and wholeness.

Contents

What Is This All About? 1
Fight! Fight! Fight! 5
Old Tapes Impede Our Ability to Make New Choices 9
Adverse Childhood Experiences (ACEs) 14
Low Self-Esteem 21
Chronic Anxiety and Depression 34
What Shall We Do With Our Hurt? 42
My Seemingly Insurmountable Impairment 51
Addictions and Pornography 56
Patterns, Generational Curses, and Family Spirits 74
Dr. Railey's Adapted Words of Encouragement 87
Scriptural Glossary 89
Acknowledgments 91
About the Author 92

What Is This All About?

Medicine and Spirituality Work Well Together

This is not a book about ghosts. It is a book about being haunted by destructive thoughts, and how to stop them.

After years of medical practice, meeting and getting to know people from all walks of life -- from criminals to heads of state, extending from poor to wealthy, I was certain of one thing: We all have problems. Some less than others; some deeply seated and sinister; while others are relatively straight forward.

Your problem could be a bad habit you fell into. It could be something you inherited through your family. Your problem could be your family. Maybe you were influenced by an adverse event. Is it possible that you want to feel good and you just haven't made good choices?

Medicine and Spirituality

My belief is that in order to achieve optimal health, the western and spiritual must be combined - meaning both the seen and the unseen must be intertwined. The ultimate in health is to combine emotional, physical, and mental health, coupled with spiritual health. Without the spiritual component, there is an incompleteness.

God has given us healthcare management for ourselves, but we've had difficulty merging the two. In certain cultures, the Spirit man was the medical man as well. Yet, over time, the Spirit man went over there and the medical man another direction... it's time to fix that.

My medical specialty for over 44 years was Family and Community Medicine… In that capacity, I was able to treat and minister to each family member instead of just singularly being a pediatrician, obstetrician or gynecologist. I wanted to be able to speak to each family member, and be able to address factors which may have gone beyond the diagnosis.

Often there was too much family dysfunction to have everyone in the same room at the same time, so I had to separate them. I learned about the big bags of chips, the two liter bottles of soda each day or the number of cigarettes truly being smoked.

A large part of my practice was using my personality as part of therapy. I would listen and learn about my patients' interests. One in particular shared a love of chess. Once we started talking about it, he stopped resisting his appointments and showed up willingly. It was always meaningful to me to see a patient light up during conversations, and mutually shared interests. I would go so far as to say connection is one of the most powerful ways to achieve healing.

I also performed minor surgeries and dealt with 'sensitive issues' which deserved greater understanding and empathy. One husband complained about his sexual relationship with his wife. Fortunately, I had already examined her and was able to inform him, with her consent that she had a physical issue concerning her uterus; it was unusual and she was extremely embarrassed about it. They had been married for 50 years and his expectations of her hadn't really changed - but they needed to because of her condition.

After speaking with them individually and privately, they were able to be supportive of each other's needs and come to some resolution. It wasn't perfect, but it gave them the space to connect and work through the challenges. Interacting in situations like this helped each to understand what was happening in the family circle.

While I didn't out rightly say it during appointments, I used my faith in God and belief in God's Word and promises to guide my mind and training to restore healing whenever possible. Inclusive of medicine, was my ability to unify families, and hopefully make a difference on a few occasions. In this work, I am boldly stating, YES, Spirituality through the Word as given in the Bible allows us to affect healing.

With understanding and practical use, we can see that God provides answers for all problems through his Word and the Holy Spirit of God. Even though the Bible may initially be cumbersome to approach, there are various versions you can read, which will help you understand in a simple manner. God didn't intend for His instructions to be complicated. He told us to be temperate in all things - which means don't go off the deep end or be extreme. Just like you don't have to exercise 7 days a week --- 20 or 30 minutes five days a week works well.

Changing the Routine

I wholeheartedly believe if you were willing to trust God, you could uncover a better version of yourself. I do lean firmly on spiritual based solutions, and encourage traditional medical interventions when appropriate.

Self-exploration, discovery and personal intervention to save yourself is very gratifying. Feeling good about yourself is also healing and joyful.

Let's fight to free ourselves from self-destructive influences.

Fight! Fight! Fight!

There's a battle in progress. It's time for you to take over!

As a boy growing up in an urban environment, it was not uncommon while on the playground to hear the piercing cry of someone shouting, "Fight! Fight! Fight!" The excited screams would pass from child to child and from group to group, spreading like fire in dry grass. Other children would rush to the scene of the crowd to see who was involved. I was often one of those kids. When it was another's turn, we took entertainment in witnessing the event. We wanted to observe all the ugly details, later relating the story over and over to others.

Sooner or later the fight comes to you. When you know you are in a fight, your response is very different than when you are the observer. You've got to realize you're in a fight, and you cannot afford to be a spectator. You've got to get in the fray, get involved and deal with the challenge, problem or the family curse or the bad habit you have acquired.

One of the great problems of our society is the large number of individuals who have not yet recognized that, "Fight! Fight! Fight!" has been declared over their entire life. We are all in a battle for the survival of who our creator intended us to be. And, our souls hang in the balance for the final outcome.

This is a book about running to the scene of our own conflict and providing some intervention.

The beginning point for stopping and controlling the ghosts of our past, which impede our progress and keep us from victory, is to first recognize their existence. We must acknowledge to ourselves that the battle is indeed on!

War Zone

Even when you didn't realize it, you have been pummeled about the head and body by negative images, memories, and sounds from your past, which seek to dismantle your confidence and disrupt your pathway. You can't fight a good fight until you first realize you are in a fight! Your response to the knowledge of the battle will determine your outcome. The purposes of the enemy (the enemies of God generally referred to as satan, satanic, or evil) in this spiritual battle are multiple. In this type of war, delay and immobilization are just as effective, and often better than complete elimination. Imagine yourself now in a war zone. The fighting is heavy and bodies are dropping. A wounded or immobilized soldier wreaks more havoc for his fellow soldiers who must care for him than if he had been simply removed from the battle or killed. You don't want to live your life as that wounded individual.

Consider a teacher who is performing his or her duties, giving incorrect information to the students. If this teacher continues in this manner, more and more individuals would be affected and wrongly taught. If we continue with our flaws unchecked, we are damaging not only ourselves, but also the people around us, just like that teacher.
So we have an obligation to not only fix our lives, but also prevent damage to those with whom we come into contact.

If not, evil can use us for its purposes, crippled and still on the field of battle. Recognizing this point is critical in understanding how keeping us bound with negative thoughts, actions, and behaviors disrupts God's personal plan for us and those around us; thus serving the kingdom of the enemy. I pray the contents of this book will help you free yourself of the negative thoughts, images, and habits which can steal your peace and inhibit your intimate walk with your Creator.

Courage to Change

Courage to make the necessary corrections is mandatory! Unfortunately, damaging behaviors carry a certain comfort with their use, which results in resistance to change. They don't want to let go of us. Therefore, once recognized and acknowledged, change is rarely easy and will require work.

As you read, you will begin to notice a common and recurrent thread, which will likely be the origin of personal and unresolved emotional conflicts... The break down and destruction of the family as a functioning unit. Hurt and emotionally wounded people are like small, preset time bombs going out and hurting other people. Confused people spread their confusion. Dysfunctional tendencies in relationships are self-perpetuating and even generational. Destruction of family structure leads to our annihilation from the inside out, similar to termites devouring the foundations of a home.

Solving the Problems Takes Recognizing Them

A significant portion of the problems or "ghosts," which haunt your present day life can often be found rooted in childhood and youthful experiences. Unresolved conflicts and personal interactions which were uncomfortable and even painful can leave scars on your emotions. It will be helpful to spend time carefully reviewing some of the unpleasant past events to gain understanding on how those events have affected you. In most cases, trying to bury a problem by not thinking about it only creates a deeper scar which can resurface in later relationships.

The first step in solving a problem is to first recognize that you have one.

Old Tapes Impede Our Ability to Make New Choices

The stories we tell ourselves continuously play in the background. The following true life excerpts give a glimpse of how unresolved and/or improperly managed thoughts, conflicts, personal traits and habits can "haunt us" in our lives and affect our behavior and personal outcomes.

Tamara's Low Self Esteem

It was 7:30 p.m. The movie would be starting about now. Once again, Greg was late without a call. Tamara felt her face begin to flush with anger and frustration as she imagined what excuses he would have this time. This has been going on since they began dating. He always had a reason that didn't completely sound true. She began to think she shouldn't have said anything about his drinking and smoking yesterday. He probably is mad and sulking and wants to break up. Her mind is racing with the possibility of having to start all over again, trying to find someone whom she could love and would love her in return. She began reconsidering the advice of her girlfriend who warned her that the relationship with Greg would never work.

She rationalized back then that Greg was never violent or abusive, and that he at least had a job and spent money on her. She felt the trust would come later with time. After all, love is forgiving always isn't it? Her inner voice agreed as she prepared herself once again to settle for another string of Greg's excuses. Her personal ghost chimed in, "It is better to avoid starting over again in another relationship. When you get married things will be different!" Deep down inside

Tamara didn't view herself as worthy of the best behavior from a man. Experiences she'd had as a child had robbed her of self-esteem.

James, An Esteemed Professional Still Felt Inferior

They strolled through the hallways of the hotel lobby, enjoying the rarity of not having anything else to do. James and his wife were on vacation, enjoying the plush atmosphere of a luxury hotel in Florida. As they entered the Gift Shop and scanned the shelves, it was obvious that everything was terribly expensive. An old familiar sense of discomfort came over James, and he heard a voice within his mind, whispering to him, "Put your hands in your pockets and don't touch anything, or else they will think you are stealing." He recognized the sound of his mother's voice from more than thirty years ago as they entered the J.C. Penney's store in urban St. Louis. The ghost of his past pressed on confidently through the personage of his mother as she spoke through the years, "Black children have to be careful so as not to be accused of stealing." Snapping back to reality, he looked at the unconcerned and cheerful attendant. It was obvious that his fears and anxiety over being watched were his alone. These thoughts were only in his head. For the first time, James realized he had feelings of inferiority which had not been eliminated by his success. James was being haunted by thoughts and experiences from his past!

Michael T. Railey, M.D.

Dan's Exposure, Leading to Addiction Started When He Was Young

Dan, a prominent attorney entered a convenience store to purchase an item for his family. He was accustomed to stopping by the magazine rack to peruse the cover stories. One cover caught his eye and held his attention. She was gorgeous! A young woman in a beautifully fitting swimsuit with an inviting smile seemed to stare back at him. His heart began to race as he contemplated what it would be like to meet her. A familiar voice within him seized the opportunity to goad him on, "She's smiling at you in a way that you would love to be adored. Look at that tan, her skin is so smooth." The magazine model was enticing.

It would be nice to see a smile like this every day, the attorney fantasized. In his mind, his thoughts justified his actions. As he lifted the magazine off the rack to purchase it, his inner voice haunted him. "You can look at this tonight, after the family is asleep." For many years now, Dan has lived a secret life filled with images of women from magazines, videos, and internet sites whom he has desired but will never meet. In his case throughout his childhood, exposure to "girly" magazines and the scantily clad women he was able to view fueled his curiosity. That and being around older boys in the neighborhood set him on this path. He and his friends had no idea they were on a trail that would be difficult to exit years later.

We Can Replace the Old Tapes

Like uncontrolled audio-visual tapes, these troublesome remnants from our childhood upbringing, exposures, experiences, and improper teachings, seem to automatically turn on in certain situations. Sometimes teasing us, at other times reminding us of old failures, we carry out behaviors that we know we don't like; but seem powerless to change. They speak to our level of self-esteem and play on our fears. For some people, the message they hear keeps them trapped at a level of anger or resentfulness. For others, the message could be a reminder of previous rejections from friends or loved ones, maybe something said to us as a child that stuck in our subconscious minds.

How do we heal from our childhood hurts? How can we ever fully recover from the pain of ridicule, and the anguish of self-doubt? Physical, psychological, emotional, and in many cases, sexual abuses from our past, continuously wash up on the shores of our consciousness, years later. These thoughts and mental implants, not unlike ghosts, track us through our daily lives; haunting us. These apparitions of our emotional make up can taunt us and immobilize us from our true potential destiny and our walk with God.

Our relationships with others is often impaired as a result of these influences. These perceived subconscious voices remind us of past doubts, discomforts, and failures. Why do so many of us fail at putting to rest the voices of personal failure and insecurity? Can they ever be dismissed? How do we change the tapes that play in our heads which cause us so much misery, mistrust, and misunderstanding?

We must learn to redirect control of the thoughts influencing our actions.

Believe me, there is a plan which has been authored by God for you. The voices of these negative influences left unchecked can eventually obstruct the wise counsel that God provides. Reading some portions of the text may be uncomfortable. Yet, on the other side of "uncomfortable" can be healing and peace. I truly believe that even for our most troublesome and personal problems, the Living Word of God has an answer.

I have introduced the term "ghost" as representative of an unseen apparition. In this sense it is not to be confused with the third person of the Trinity, "Holy Ghost." It is my prayer that for you the reader, that your ghost(s) will be called out and identified; and that you will learn from your own personal experience that God truly does have a solution to "stop the haunting" in your life, quieting the negative voices which can steal the peace, confidence, and contentment from your existence.

I have seen three general areas which create the greatest proportion of personal challenges. They are:

**1.) Anxiety and Depression,
2.) Low Self-esteem and;
3.) Various Addictions (food, drugs, materialism, sex).**

Although there are obviously many, many, more problems, these three will be emphasized.

It is time that you put a stop to the haunting in your life and bury the spirit of your personal ghosts, thus freeing yourself for a life of peace and fruitful living!

Adverse Childhood Experiences

Research has shown that childhood trauma can affect our health and wellbeing throughout life.

In 1997 one of the most important health related studies in recent times was revealed as a result of a collaboration between Kaiser Permanente and the Center for Disease Control (CDC). More than 17,000 individual cases were examined leading to the conclusion that genetic alterations in DNA often result from adverse childhood experiences (ACEs) such as neglect, sexual and emotional abuse, physical abuse, dysfunctional family interactions, and others.

They discovered that there is a connection between certain specific Adverse Childhood Experiences and medical outcomes. Social and mental health disorders such as depression, anxiety, violence, and criminal activities could be related to the numbers of these negative events we experience. Studies show about 67% of the U.S. population has at least one ACE. When a person has an ACE score of four or more, their life expectancy is diminished. Please review Figure 1, which lists 10 Categories for ADVERSE CHILDHOOD EXPERIENCES.

Michael T. Railey, M.D.

Figure 1:
10 Categories for Adverse Childhood Experiences

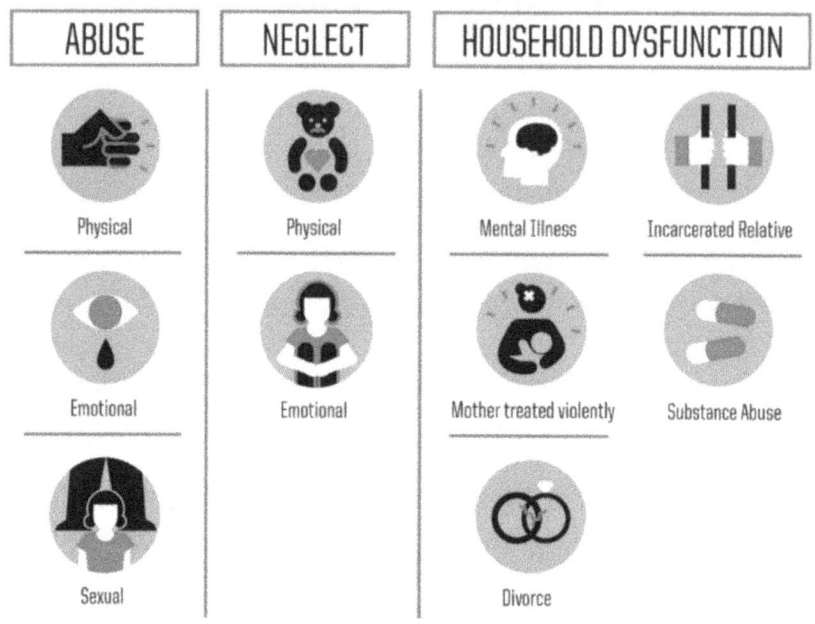

Source: Centers for Disease Control and Prevention
Credit: Robert Wood Johnson Foundation

Most people are not aware of this public health threat although the knowledge of it has been around for more than 20 years.

Though health care professionals are aware of the study, they often bypass the significance of this. Practicing medicine should include getting to root causes, and we now know with certainty that these contributors can dramatically alter the course of one's life if unaddressed.

As you review the 10 factors and Figure 1, count the number of issues you were exposed to as a child - in other words,

if you or someone in your household suffered from, was exposed to, or experienced one or more of these factors, count them up... Now that you have this information,
Do you recognize any illnesses within yourself or in your family that could be related to this problem?

Figure 2: Medical Impact of ACE'S

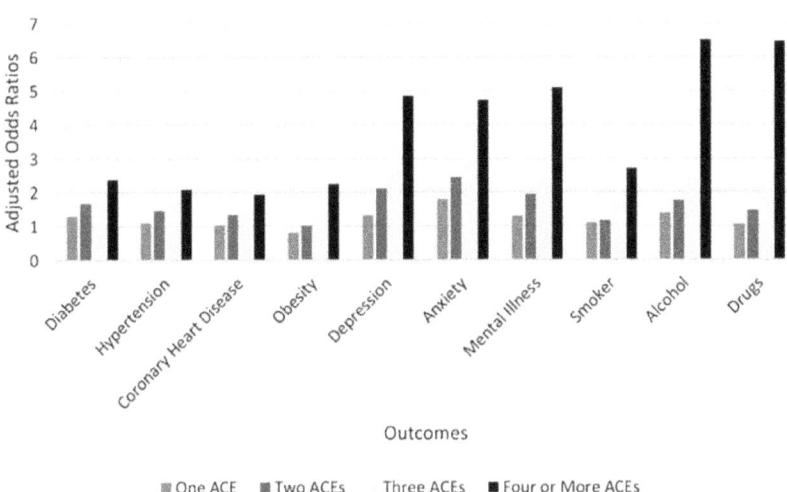

Adverse childhood experiences in association with health, mental health, and risky behavior in the kingdom of Saudi Arabia - Scientific Figure on ResearchGate.net, uploaded by Maha A. Almuneef.

Any problem that you've experienced should be screened for a potential connection to a childhood experience. *Yes! Your "problem" may be related to something from your past.* With that knowledge, you can find understanding, perhaps anger, and eventually relief now that you know you likely suffered because of things that happened to you, not necessarily because of you. So, look at it this way, the question is not always *"What is wrong with me?"* it is more, *"What happened to me?"*

Here are a few examples of Adverse Childhood Experiences as they played out in my practice and in my observations in life:

A high school teen has been teased and ridiculed both by family and school classmates because of a skin disorder causing discoloration, darkening and scarring. She also has asthma. The student is seen as quiet, withdrawn and even depressed. *Her emotional development, school performance and ability to socialize have been affected by her ACEs.*

An adult administrative assistant with severe obesity was diagnosed with diabetes. She lived in many foster homes throughout her life until she aged out at 19, as she was never adopted. *Her emotional development and eating habits have been affected by her ACEs.*

A teenager, who became pregnant, was discovered to have suffered neglect, sexual abuse, and low self-esteem throughout late childhood. Her mother had a similar history and pregnancy when she was sixteen. *Her efforts and desire to feel loved has contributed to her early pregnancy and self-image issues.*

A thirty year old with minor physical injury, has a long history of traffic tickets and fighting. He suffered physical and emotional abuse in his household as a child, and has a long record of incarceration and becoming a bully himself. *He became who he was as a result of what he experienced.*

It is important to understand the greater the number of ACES and depth of microtrauma, (trauma often experienced, but unseen) the greater emotional, physical, and mental stress, in most cases.

Consider Your Life and Influences

With this information, the pathway to your recovery must also take into account what happened to you during the process of healing. It gives you the power to make new choices as you work to counteract the challenges you've been facing.

When we consider mental and emotional problems which could "haunt us" into adulthood, it is vital to consider adverse childhood experiences as potential root causes.

Not everyone who experiences a negative childhood event suffers damage. Depending upon the emotional make up and support system of each child, many may have no harm done. But, it is certainly impossible to predict what microtrauma will do to each person in advance.

I distinctly recall growing up in my neighborhood where nicknames were assigned to an individual according to his or her physical appearance. The casual reference of a playmate to a friend as having an odd shaped head could lead to a demeaning time of being referred to as "peanut or peanut head" by class members.

One child may take this with a laugh and another could be seriously embarrassed and feel insecure for years. Certainly, there are far worse experiences a child could suffer, but we never know the depth of pain and reaction that could occur. One circumstance might encourage an individual to great accomplishments, while another may evolve into the class bully to protect their personal esteem and strike first.

Spend some time reviewing and considering the charts provided and try to recall if you and/or someone close to you has experienced any of these. Remembering the first step to recovery is generally recognition. By exposing our past pains to the light of understanding and forgiveness, we begin our own personal past to healthier emotions and minimize sources of stress.

Take Aways

There are three primary ways to address the problems of Adverse Childhood Experiences.

1. **Trauma Informed Care** - often done on a pediatric doctor level, children can be evaluated and treated in order to lessen the potential effects in the future.

2. **Trauma Informed Counseling** - from professionals who can relate to your adult circumstances and support you in processing and moving through the behaviors and patterns which may still be affecting you.

3. **Seeking a Strong Spiritual Connection** - through attending spiritual services, reading scripture and fellowshipping with others of like-mindedness, research has proven this method is effective, as an additive to the above two.

The ACEs evaluation and treatment for these conditions is available; however, it's not widely promoted as this work takes resources, coordination and a commitment to "do the work." Economics along with racial and ethnic barriers have been factors in limiting the "system" from broadly treating individuals and families in this manner. I encourage you to use the internet to take an ACEs evaluation and to seek a center or professional who could support you and your family in working through these factors.

The first and most important thing you can do is to have a reliable, steady person in your life who does not repeat nuisances of the experiences that happened to you.

Low Self-Esteem

Low self-esteem can be overcome by the acquisition and usage of a set of skills.

Those skills are gradually built upon and enlarged as we obtain an accurate picture of ourselves. The negative tapes that have played in the minds of the Angie, Maria, John and Lois have roots in reduced self-worth. They consistently settle because "that's what they've always done." They don't know what's happening in order to replace the tapes. You'll likely recognize some of the choices and outcomes in their stories, and be able to relate on some level. The good news? *Low self-esteem can be changed with sincere, focused effort.*

It is mandatory to discover your gift or gifts of the Holy Spirit and use them to serve God. This along with other specifics which follow will lead to a new confidence and eradication of personal low self-esteem and the destructive patterns it generates.

The things that have led you into negative situations and high stress should also be monitored such as inappropriate spending and purchases, misuse of time, bad eating, and drinking habits as well. Discovering and maintaining strong self-esteem is work that requires fitness and feeling good about yourself.

Let's explore:

_____

Fat Angie

The class reunion was now a week away. Angie had not lost the weight she had intended to lose. As she looked in the mirror at herself, she could hear the voices of her past outside of the fifth grade classroom. The boys were huddled together as they made fun of her, "Fat Angie is your girlfriend!" one boy teased. The boy responded with anger at the suggestion of what had become the supreme insult and class joke. The pain of overhearing that ridicule had never left her subconscious. This was in addition to the teasing she received on a regular basis from her brothers and sisters. As time went on, Angie found safety in staying to herself, and avoiding public places and events where she could be seen. The inner voice, which haunted her, reassured her that going to the reunion would be a mistake as she was so unsightly, ugly, and fat.

Maria's Mom Set the Tone

Since childhood, Maria never seemed to excel at anything that she thought was really important. She was actually very attractive and even beautiful by most standards. In her mind, she considered herself nothing special, and she carried herself accordingly. A closer look into her background revealed an only child who was constantly criticized by her mother. Her mother was uncomfortable with her daughter's attractiveness; having low self-esteem herself. She sought to control her daughter by reminding her of mediocrity and teasing her with anticipated failures in her endeavors. Maria had a very poor self-concept, didn't believe in her talents and didn't understand why men were attracted to her. As the years rolled by, she would fall into sexual relationships with men she later discovered she should have avoided. Having assigned little or no value to her many undiscovered attributes, she often settled for much less in life than she could have and should have. This was a pattern that dominated the first three or four decades of her life and changed her very destiny.

_____

John's Thick Glasses

The contact lens was torn! It was after 6:00 p.m. and the eye doctor's office was closed. John quickly considered his options when the voice of his buried self-esteem spoke out. "How many fingers?" his ghost laughed. Suddenly, he could see the faces and hear the crowd of children standing about him as his inquisitor waived fingers frantically in front of his face. The other children were poised to burst into laughter as they watched and waited for his response. Another child exclaimed, "You can't see nothin' without those coke bottles! Man, are you blind!" The voices from his past sneered at him as the children cackled with glee. Forcing himself back to the present, John quickly decided it would be better to wear only one lens and take his chances driving than to risk the pain of more ridicule and jesting from anyone at the business meeting he was scheduled to attend in an hour. John remained ashamed of his poor vision and thick glasses. This had affected his self-confidence throughout his childhood influencing his social life and his self-esteem, and remains with him as an adult.

_____

Loose Lois

Lois, a 29-year-old secretary with a large company admits that she doesn't understand her own actions. She knew that Ronnie was not the man of her dreams. He smoked and occasionally drank too much. Ronnie was seldom, if ever, thoughtful and loving to her. He didn't do those little special things that many women love so much. He was often late or didn't call appropriately when he delayed in meeting her. Recently, she discovered he smoked marijuana routinely, and occasionally inhaled cocaine. Nevertheless, she had fallen into a sexual relationship with him, and the relationship has continued for years. She felt that marriage was out of the question, and even described him as not being "marriage material." Her ghost spoke what seemed to be good logic. "At least you have a man. After all, nobody is perfect."

Lois, like many other women today, felt compelled to give herself away, spending her precious intimacy, a gift of God, in a dead end relationship. As a child, Lois had been sexually molested and could not rationalize her acts of low self-esteem and the relationship between her past and her current behavior. She had never observed how a respectful man treats a woman with love and with commitment. She had not seen it demonstrated nor experienced it. Lois had very little contact with her biological father and certainly no relationship with him over the years.

In order to develop a successful, personal relationship, Lois will have to hold herself in high enough esteem to not allow substandard treatment. Our world is full of men who prey on women like Lois; using and discarding them at will.

Michael T. Railey, M.D.

Recognizing the Problems and Patterns

Can you relate? If so, perhaps someone you know, or yourself, is suffering with low self-esteem. I believe a major contributor to poor self-esteem is dysfunctional families and the evolution of increased divorce rates. In today's society, divorce has become so common that we have mistakenly de-emphasized the tremendous damage that comes out of broken relationships and forced single parenting. There are many parents who do a fine job of raising their children alone, but having both parents in place remains God's preferred way.

Moses, considered a great patriarch of the Bible, was the powerful figure who led the Israelites out of slavery. Yet, even Moses was at one time doubtful of his abilities and very hesitant to carry out God's command on his life. Moses had a speech impediment which contributed to his self-esteem problem. God finally settled the issue as he grew aggravated with Moses and his excuses for disobedience, by allowing his brother Aaron to go with him and speak for him. The great Moses who parted the Red Sea fearlessly was initially afraid to stand before the Pharoah of Egypt with Gods' commands and instruction, without his brother Aaron by his side. *Moses unbelief and esteem problems were not explained, as is often the case with many of us today.*

Angie, Maria, John and Lois' reduced self-worth and their lack of knowledge of how to repair their underdeveloped confidence is personally devastating and generationally infectious. How we feel about ourselves is determined by a number of significant influences. The most important of which is that influence of our family members and particularly our parents, who serve as our main source of nurturing, and a mirror of how we can be seen by others. Family influences that are negative position us for a lifetime battle of uphill struggling, striving for recovery of normal feelings about ourselves. Children who are missing parental input from two sources speculate at what "normality" might be, and often guess wrongly. Today men often guess at what being a man really means as they have not had a close up and personal role model.

Change Makers Have Often Suffered Trauma

When you are one of the people in your family who breaks the cycles and changes things, you will almost certainly have had trauma in childhood. This has happened because satan does not know what you're going to do, but knows *the Lord is focusing on you!* So, satan tries to mess with you… You can take that as good news --- Some are put in place to save the family, alter the pathways, shift the negative habits/traditions, and will have the ability to bail things out…

For the larger portion of his early life, Moses didn't know his true identity; he didn't know his family nor why he had been placed into an adoptive family. It was only when God gave him instruction, direction and purpose for his life, did he become the Moses remembered triumphantly.

Is Low Self-Esteem A Problem?

If you sense a lack of confidence with your daily endeavors and are afraid to take chances which could lead to bettering your life and welfare, you very well may suffer from low self-esteem. Other examples include those of us who doubt our physical attributes and are extremely unhappy with our body build or even our intelligence. You would be surprised at the numbers of professionals I have met with, who admit privately that they secretly fear being revealed as "phonies," or who fear being "discovered" as incompetent. Adults with a history of physical, sexual, and or psychological abuse are also a set up for a future of low self-esteem. Some of these situations require extensive counseling with trained professionals. Each of us can also benefit from the teachings of Jesus Christ. His words provide us with extensive help and intervention to assist us through the counseling of the Holy Spirit of God to help us regain healthy personal esteem.

Solutions

1. Recognition is usually the first step for correction of any problem. We only attempt to fix that which we recognize as broken. Be true to yourself and accept your doubtfulness about your abilities and/or your appearance as proof positive of the existence of a problem, which can be fixed. Now that you are aware of the way Adverse Childhood Experiences can affect us, consider the risk factors including childhood bullying, ridicule, and insufficient encouragement. Consider the negative factors which may have encompassed your experiences. If there was no counterbalance or few positive support systems provided, many of the feelings and behaviors experienced "make sense."

We are instructed to, "Trust in the Lord with all thine heart and lean not unto thine own understanding. In all thy ways acknowledge him and he shall direct thy path." (Proverbs 3:5-6). *Stop here and re-read the two sentences.* Dwell here long enough to remember and memorize this short, but vital passage.

It will be vital to you in your life over and over again. *At the root of most low self-esteem situations are problems in development of appropriate basic trust.* **People who can't trust are afraid to venture out into new arenas.** The risk of failure at new relationships or undertakings creates greater fear and trepidation than that created with individuals not having this problem. Being fearful to risk change can even impair your relationship with God, as God requires trust (faith) from his followers in all situations. Hebrews 11:6 states, "But without faith it is impossible to please him: for he that cometh to God must believe that he is, and that he is a rewarder of them that diligently seek him." When a person finds him/herself in circumstances whereby they cannot trust any fleshly beings in life, the chances of trusting an invisible spirit being are very minimal.

I have a colleague who is an excellent physician, but has experienced lifelong mental blocks believing in the one true God because of the bad relationship she experienced with her natural father. Her lack of basic trust in men started with him, and has affected her entire life. This has become a common problem for many.

This basic trust is desired by God of us towards Him. **However, it starts in childhood with learning to trust loved ones and obtaining love in return.** A major task therefore for a person of low self-esteem is to learn to trust God and his promises above all else.

2. Set about the task of discovering your spiritual gifts with the help of private prayer, pastoral input, close friends or loved ones. Review your past circumstances in life. This will help you figure out where you were designed to fit in the kingdom of God in terms of your function. People who have been around you and hopefully care for you over the years have observed your behavior and have certain thoughts about you. If you are picking a gift that is in your mind glamourous but is not the truth of who you are, your loved ones can be a filter for you. And in the same way, people who know you can agree with it if the picture you place on yourself is accurate, as you've probably been doing it all along.

The Holy Bible says that every person who accepts Christ as his or her Savior has at least one gift. Most have several gifts. When you use your spiritual gifts in your everyday life, your very existence begins to feel more justified and your self-worth is automatically more complete. It is the individual who does not use his/her gift(s) out of ignorance who experience difficulty recognizing God's intent for their life. Therefore, those who have discovered their "spiritual" gifts don't harbor low self-esteem. They instead develop assurance that whatever they don't have was not intended; so as to make room for what they do have in terms of capabilities. There are many gifts of a spiritual nature, and they range from knowledge, discernment, hospitality, and teaching; to prophesy, mercy, giving, and healing. Read about gifts in 1 Corinthians Chapter 12 of the Bible. Membership in a Bible teaching and a believing church under the shepherding of a Godly inspired Pastor can help you discover your place within the body of Christ.

3. Be cautious in considering marriage until issues of personal esteem have been addressed and corrected, as people who have low self-esteem are usually incapable of making truly accurate relationship evaluations. Much like an individual who is colorblind, people can unknowingly miss important characteristics and misjudge observations until self-esteem is intact. *Women and men of low self-esteem are particularly prone to be fooled by self-serving godless mates until esteem issues are corrected and discerning abilities are intact.*

4. Create a personal diary and make regular entries about episodes of distress, your feelings, and what happens as a result. Over time you'll be able to review your progress and notice that likely, your patterns are changing and so are the outcomes. When this happens, you'll be able to exchange hopelessness for hope.

5. Create a vision for you and write it down. Having a plan for what you want in your life and thinking big will assist you in achieving it. Then match your desires to the word of God's teachings. God, in answer to your prayers, will provide you those things, which serve His kingdom and its purposes. Be prepared to make appropriate commitments and do the work required to realize the goals you have realistically set for yourself. Don't forget to write those out as well.

6. Pray that God will restore you to a level of wellness and confidence. Additionally, pray for receiving Godly persons into your life for you to interact with and provide you with wise counsel. Those of us on the path of recovery need to "Walk not in the counsel of the ungodly (Psalm 1)."

You should associate and affiliate with people who make you feel good about yourself. Changing people, places, and things will assist you in growth and development. Places you may have frequented where negative people and conditions are abundant should also be avoided. Seek out organizations and groups filled with positive thinking memberships and activities. You've heard the saying, "birds of a feather flock together."

7. Courageously go after ways of strengthening your confidence by developing physical fitness and good health. Proper exercise and nutritional management goes a long way towards maintaining an environment which is conducive to success and confidence. Our physical bodies are temples to God and the Holy Spirit. God in His wise creation of us has given us a physiological system which responds to exercise with an outpouring of specific chemicals which tends to relax and have an anti-anxiety affect. *If your temple (body) is corrupted with cigarettes, various drugs, alcohol, poor nutrition, and sexual promiscuity your thought processes and energy level will be affected and even surely significantly diminished (1 Corinthians 6:19, Romans 12:1).*

8.   Regardless of your past, when it comes to your self-worth and service to God, all prior experiences can be worked out for good and for God's plan (Romans 8:28). History is filled with successful people of God with difficult and even sordid past lives, having participated in everything from drug abuse and prostitution to political corruption and moral degradation. These people are still children of God. When you ask the LORD for mercy, grace and endurance, sincerely, He joins the battle. With daily repetition, meditation, and study, you will strengthen your spiritual muscles and resolve as you build your personal relationship with Him.

9.   Seek out and find involvement in a Bible believing, Bible teaching church where leadership is Christ centered and pastored by a sincere and humble leader. People of past low self-esteem, seeking restoration, require proper teaching and leadership for recovery and trust to develop. (Hebrews 10:25). Always seek to find what I've described, and do not settle for insincerity or lack of spiritual uplift.

10.   Study, understand and memorize, as many promises of God as you can find with reading and research. Your hopes, dreams, and your self-esteem rest on the promises of God. The foremost promise being that of your salvation through Christ. Your place in eternity rests upon your acceptance of Christ as your personal savior.

When you truly convince yourself of this and not just take the words as trite sayings, then you will be well on your way to redeveloping the esteem of a saved and redeemed child of God -- a person of confidence and wholeness, and an individual who takes risks and survives failures without fear.

Going through an exit allows you to step into a new entrance.

Chronic Anxiety and Depression

Long spells of sadness or nervousness can lead to serious consequences.

I once heard a somewhat amusing story about the devil having a garage sale. It was reported almost everything available had been sold except one odd shaped object hanging on the wall. Potential buyers asked what it was and the price. Each time satan stated flatly that was not for sale – "It is my most useful tool."

Finally, one potential buyer pushed back until a more complete answer was given. Satan explained, "You see that's not for sale because it is my most useful tool. It is discouragement and depression. When I can keep my customer depressed, they lose hope. And, when hopeless, my work is nearly done. Hopelessness leads to ineffectiveness and no desire to strive for anything to change their situation."

This 'story' points out a significant fact we need to recognize. Hopelessness defeats the human spirit and desire to fight. Without the desire and energy to resist negative thinking and thoughts, we cannot regain God's path for our lives. We can become like a ship without a rudder, wandering aimlessly to and from wrong thoughts and behaviors until we ultimately waste our lives and/or end our existence.

That is the reason there are so many references to thought and thought management in the Bible. We are what we think about.

We must learn to trap un-useful and improper thinking as soon as we recognize it is happening, and redirect it. We must not dwell on past events; instead, we must choose to move on to better outcomes.

Anxiety

Anxiety, worry, and depressive disorders are common to all of us at some point in time in our lives. For many people, depression and nervous anxieties become a way of life. Any glimmer of hope they see is soon brushed away by a pervasive sadness which overtakes them. They eventually expect to fail at most things they attempt. For some, suicide begins to appear as an almost logical solution. For others the "slow suicide" of alcoholism, drugs, cigarette smoking, or overeating yields temporary relief for an otherwise hopeless situation. Depression is one of the most common mental disorders in primary health care settings. 20 percent of women and 10 percent of men experience this problem. Depression is a major cause of death. Between 30,000 and 40,000 Americans commit suicide each year.

Anxiety is often rooted in childhood experiences where confusion and uncertainty presents in familial patterns of depression from generation to generation, childhood experiences and in particular, unstable unpredictable childhood experiences often serve as a precursor to anxiety in adulthood. The actual quantity of genetic influence leading to the manifestation of adult anxiety is unknown, but clearly significant with increased risk of anxiety developing if one or both parents experienced the condition.

Sad and Anxious Lonnie

Lonnie has been nervous since she could remember. The term "gets on my nerves", was her frequent phrase. It seemed that the little things bothered her to a greater extent than others. Any problem with a family member or a close friend felt personal to her, and she seemed to worry about some of everything. It was so bad that reading or hearing about certain criminal acts could make her nervous. If an illness developed, she always expected the worst. One summer she noticed a bump on her forearm. She thought she recalled a bug bite after working in her garden. It seemed to itch a lot and she scratched it often. Her "personal ghost" encouraged her insecurities with, *This could be skin cancer. You know you've always suspected you would get it.* Lonnie neglected to make a doctor's appointment because she feared the diagnosis. As she nervously and unconsciously scratched and picked at the small sore twenty or thirty times a day, it began to get darker and scaly in appearance. The voice of her anxiety said, *Why did this have to happen to you. When the cancer is diagnosed you'll need an amputation. Extreme? Yes. "Real" to Lonnie? Unfortunately, yes. Worrying over every little thing and propelling yourself into a frenzy of negativity can lead to depression and chronic anxiety.*

Hopeless Cal

It all seemed so hopeless now. Just as it has been in the past, Cal felt as if the bottom of his life was dropping out. He knew the number of layoffs on his job were increasing, and any day he could be terminated. His marital situation wasn't much better. Karen and Cal seemed to be on different wave lengths for every topic. Even a casual conversation led to an argument. It was as if they couldn't please each other anymore with anything. It didn't help that he was gaining weight. His personal confidence was at an all-time low. Even playing cards with the guys once a month was not as much fun anymore. He felt like a black cloud followed him at all times. Cal thought about taking his own life. His ghost agreed with him, You are better off dead. *Your family will have more cash available and lead a better life after you are gone.* Church seemed to be a waste of time. He felt that the Pastor's words weren't for him, and that no one understood his deep sorrow. Never one to talk much, Cal didn't have any close friends with whom he felt comfortable sharing with. His ghost had Cal boxed in. Planning for suicide was his next serious consideration. *Isolation can be dangerous.*

Crying Cassandra

Cassandra could feel her face turning red as the tears welled up in her eyes. Maybe it was a little thing to others, but it was big to her. Jim had forgotten their anniversary again. You would think after seven years he would remember - she always did. It was the same thing yesterday when he neglected to open the door for her. Jim said she cried about something every day. She couldn't even understand it herself. She couldn't sleep well and her appetite was lousy. After missing breakfast and lunch, the thought of food was almost nauseating. She felt empty, hollow even, as if someone had carved out her insides with a big knife.

A voice within subtly hinted, You'll never be happy. Quitting your job and having a stay at home Mom was the worst mistake you could've ever made. She couldn't stop the tears. *There are likely several factors contributing to Cassandra's feelings of depression.*

My Own Experiences with Anxiety

In my life I have been blessed by not experiencing a major depression requiring intervention and medication. I believe my love of sports and connections with spiritually based groups and organizations has protected me to a great extent. This has not been the case with anxiety. For the greater portion of my life, I have struggled with generalized and performance anxiety to an almost crippling degree. From attending a social event and dating to making a presentation or an athletic performance, I was often nearly overwhelmed with gastric distress, trembling, and panic attacks.

In the neighborhoods I have lived, the presence of bullies and their families was common. Being assaulted by one or more persons comes to my memory on at least four separate occasions. Fortunately, I was never seriously injured or physically hurt. For many years, I surveyed shadows around me and checked over my shoulders to prevent attack from the rear. In my adult life, there has not been anyone there, but I remained vigilant. The fear and dread of experiencing an event which has not materialized is one of the major distinguishing manifestations of anxiety.

The body goes into a hypervigilant mode to prepare to run and escape, or fight. There are multiple types of anxieties but I won't try and describe them all, here.

Depression characterized by low mood generally involves a loss or diminished enjoyment in the elements of every day life. It manifests in sleep patterns, eating habits, recreational changes and potentially sexual behaviors.

Angela, a usually vibrant computer analyst and athlete complains of gradual changes after the passing of her husband Phil. They had been together for over 30 years and did practically everything together. Although Phil's passing was not unexpected, Angela seemed to be unable to regain her desire to jog, read, and do community service. Their children were unsuccessful in consoling her. *Some people have situational depression related to an event, and others develop depression from no apparent cause.*

Without intervention, many become "haunted" by a spirit of depression. "I might as well be dead," a voice from within seems to say. "You will never be the same and you are only a burden now."

Know this: The Holy Spirit of God **never** reminds us of our failures, but responds to our declarations of imperfection with grace and mercy through forgiveness and positive encouragement.

When the symptoms of mood changes and depression occur consistently over a more than two weeks without relief, the diagnosis of a major depression can be considered. It is beyond the scope of this book to go into any depth of describing the large numbers of medications that are used to treat the various types of depressions. However, it is important to note that mild and moderate depression can often be managed without the intervention of medicines. Consultation with a physician can assist in sorting out severity.

Fortunately, the suggestions offered here are beneficial no matter how severe the problem. Recognizing that our mood changes accompanied by sleep problems, appetite changes, increasing or decreasing sexual desire, and a lack of pleasure in participating in previously joyful activities must be recognized as suggestive of a significant mood disorder. Thinking that these feelings will dissipate or go away on their own can be a big mistake. It never hurts to discuss your thoughts with a close friend or relative, and consider what has been happening in your life currently or in the past, that could be contributing. If the problems you have noted have been going on for two or more weeks, make a medical appointment and begin your own interventions to address this challenge.

1. Notify a few close friends and/or relatives of your need for prayer and checking with you as you deal with this challenge. Make some appointments for coffee, tea or a meal on several days.

2. Review and memorize Biblical scriptures such as Phil 4:6-10 and Romans 8:28 to remind you to focus your thoughts. You have promised security through your belief system and the Word of God. Try to get to and maintain hopefulness and gratefulness for what you do have. Write this down and review frequently. You are creating a human bio-computer chip to rely upon as you press through and fight anxiety.

3. Exercise is actually an antidepressant and is also calming for anxiety. There are studies revealing that approximately 30 minutes of exercise at least four times per week is as effective as medications in managing mild to moderate depression.

Severe depression as determined by a medical professional often results in the use of prescription medications.

Exercising regularly and consistently whether "depressed or anxious" is a great practice for us all.

> *"Your body is the temple...so glorify God in your body."*
> *- 1 Corinthians 6:19-20*

What Shall We Do With Our Hurt?

I have been fortunate to maintain contact on a continuous basis with a few colleagues who are still in active practice. This has been particularly useful in keeping me abreast of many mood disturbances and related complaints which represent today's state of mind. In addition to the general need of addressing mental illness problems there seems to be an increase in "offences or personal hurt" from our daily interactions at home, work, and with relationships. This warranted, I felt a need to tell a personal story which happened during my youth that changed me considerably, and has taken many decades to work through. In fact, I can easily state the situation "haunted" me throughout my career, and I have only recently put it to rest!

I use this story as an example of how an unresolved negative incident can have continuous smoldering effects on our lives, often without us being aware of it.

What do we do with the hurt when nobody's apologizing for what they did or what happened?

The Fall of 1975

To the best of my recollection, it was the first time (hopefully the only time) in my adult life that I would consider a plot to eliminate another person. The surgical resident for the month, let's call him Dr. P., had embarrassed me openly at the nurses' station in a way I felt was totally uncalled for and certainly inappropriate.

Michael T. Railey, M.D.

I could feel the eyes of the other medical team members observing for my reactions as the resident angrily exclaimed, "Where else do you think it could be?" He referred to the placement of a plastic suction catheter I had attempted to place in the stomach of a distressed patient. He continued to scream at me as I cowered within, uncertain of what to say or to do in this situation. He was the senior resident on my surgical rotation, and the word among the African American medical students who preceded me was that the surgery rotation would be our most severe challenge. Was it my fate to become another statistic by failing, dropping out or being dismissed?

I was a new third year medical student, wet behind the ears and afraid that the nasogastric catheter I had placed was in an incorrect position. The patient seemed too uncomfortable to me, and had coughed multiple times. As I tried to explain my specific actions to him, Dr. P. stomped away from the nursing station and into the patient's room as I followed meekly. Once in the room, he selected a 30 cc plastic syringe and injected air rather rapidly into the tube while we listened to the area between the chest wall and the stomach wall. The whoosh of air I heard through my stethoscope confirmed that I had placed the tube correctly. My patient's level of anxiety subsided as I taped the catheter down to secure it while simultaneously trying to reassure the patient in spite of my embarrassed state.

No further problems with the nasogastric tube occurred, but even after patient discharge, my ears continued to burn with embarrassment. None of the other students spoke with me or attempted to console me that day. I felt isolated and disrespected. Much later, one of my fellow students told me the questions I had been asked on rounds were questions he did not know how to answer.

That conversation helped me to feel more justified in my position - but it didn't change my feelings about Dr. P.

It was apparent to me by Dr. P.'s management of the situation which occurred, his general management of the surgical residents, and his treatment of me throughout the entire rotation, that he held me in low regard both as a student and as a human being. At no point in time during the one month rotation did he seek to teach me anything, but instead seemed to revel in selecting questions I did not know the answer to whenever possible. Whenever I did respond with a correct response, he demanded to know how I knew the answer and why I answered as I had. It seemed to be a no win situation no matter what. I had no idea of what to do and feared reporting this to any attending physician, as I was totally intimidated. I thought how sweet the world might be if he never existed or if by some miracle he could be eliminated. Fortunately, my feelings of needing revenge were overwhelmed by the possibilities of the many legal consequences I would have to live through, if I acted on my anger and frustration.

My experiences on that rotation left me with a bad feeling towards considering surgery as my specialty. Many of us felt that some specialties we were just not welcome to participate in, and the effort to swim against the current was not worth difficulties, obstacles and bias. Although I had never written of the incident until now, the event had a profound effect on my psychological state and confidence, from which I would not recover for decades.

Over the course of the next year, many other incidents were experienced by me and other African American students. Most of them I heard about after the fact, years later. Whenever we physicians gathered privately, many stories would be shared of mistreatment, poor evaluations, and intimidation. I am certain many non-minority students could tell their share of stories as well. But for Black students later to become physicians and supervisory physicians ourselves, I believe most of us would battle internally over whether it was really our knowledge deficit which led to our harsh treatment or the fact we were Black. I have since spoken with many now prominent academicians, teachers, attending physicians, faculty members, and private minority doctors who seem to go into a near hypnotic state as they discuss the painful experiences they lived through, and the sense of injustice encountered.

We knew that many of our colleagues felt we didn't belong, and/or that we shouldn't even be in medical school. That didn't help things. Regardless of the motives in our assailant's minds, it was the processing of these experiences over and over again that wore us down and kept us with constant feelings of stress and inferiority during our young years of development. We now know that post traumatic stress disorders (PTSD) certainly can spring from experiences like these. Of the seven African Americans initially in my medical school class, I was the only one of us to graduate on time.

I have since lost contact with all of the others for various reasons. For sure, we would be unlikely to meet at any of the reunions. For most of my adult career, I thought *Why would the prisoner who escaped, return to his cell voluntarily?* I believe we all wanted to forget our years at the school and just put it all behind us.

When I departed from the University as a graduate new physician looking ahead to post graduate training, I could not imagine wanting to ever return to my medical school.

Certainly there was no love in me at that time for my experience or the people associated with the school. My greatest regret is all of the friends and associates I could have had. I didn't reach out and neither did they. I know now that we were not normal ourselves in the state of paranoia in which we lived.

One day we found written on the blackboard in our small classroom, *"Just because you are paranoid doesn't mean someone is NOT out to get you!"* We all laughed uncomfortably. Yet, for me and my associates, it was a truth. Medical school and training was not a normal time in my life.

Fifty years have passed since graduation, and in my capacity as a member of the Dean's staff and an associate professor at a different University but same state, I've spoken with many students, residents, and some faculty who've had similar experiences.

One day a new fledgling African American attending and I were discussing med school experiences. Her eyes became glazed over as if she had been suddenly teleported through time and was re-experiencing the past all over again. She spoke of what she felt was discriminatory infractions committed against her and the pain she still recalled from her experience. Parts of this conversation were identical with many black students, now physicians whom I have met over the years.

It was then that I asked myself, *What shall we do with our pain? Can we place it on a shelf and forget about it? Does it hang about our necks like a noose, needing only the tug of a memory to tighten? Where does anyone go with their past mistreatments that can never be corrected?*

How can we let it go and move on in a healthy manner? Why should we?

I have posed a lot of questions, but one thing for certain is that holding on to the past will not change anything and seldom does anyone or anything good. **In fact whether a wrong was ever forgiven or not, justified or not; the holder of the unforgiveness suffers continuously from their own unforgiveness.** It is like an insidious hidden wound which left unchecked only festers, drains, and continues to rage.

For me, although the memories shall remain forever, I chose not to re-taste the bitterness inflicted upon me by those who sought to hurt me either by purpose or by accident. I would like to see my classmates who I didn't get to know. I would like to greet them with a smile instead of with disguised pain.

Even though you may not have been in medical training, think of a time in your life when you've been hurt unnecessarily or treated inappropriately. These situations are difficult to let go of - but very damaging to hold on to.

So, let us step away from the emotion of those moments and do that which we need to do to help us to heal and move on.

The first step of recovery from any loss or death is **Denial** - We can't believe this (event) has happened to us.

Second is **Anger** - That we were subjected to it or that it even happened!

The third major step is **Acceptance**. Only by moving past anger can we go on to acceptance and gain a healthy perspective.

In medicine, we define *pathologic grief* as grieving which remains unresolved for six months or more. We don't need an outside consultation to determine that; if we don't do something to close our wounds we become locked in pathologic grief, doctor, patient or not.

Further, this certainly doesn't do honor to those who came before us in American history, and suffered far greater overt injustices than we've ever had to bare.

So how can we facilitate the passing of our anger? For me, I have resigned myself joyfully to the fact that I chose to apply to the school I applied to, and they chose to accept me. If these two choices do not occur, I am without the dream of my lifetime to become a physician. That is really what counts and that is an opportunity that not everyone gets! It is up to me to make the best of my life as it stands with the MD behind my name as my title.

No matter what I went through - I earned it. The Bible says in James that we should "count it all joy" when we fall or when we are subject to divers temptations (hurdles/obstacles). He reminds us to let the event work its purpose on us to create patience and endurance, which leads to completeness.

When we feel betrayed, we must get past our pain and hurt by realizing that what 'they' may have meant for bad, God allowed for good. If we do not allow the process to be finished, we lose a portion of our completeness, which is not God's desire for our lives and purpose. We should rejoice in the strength of our victories against any mistreatment we might have received as making us stronger.

Finally, we are commanded to forgive and not asked to

forgive. By doing so, we set a precedent for forgiveness in our own lives. Believe it or not, we will offend someone at some time in our own lives and maybe not even realize it!

Let us return to the places that we've avoided, finding our rewards and renewal. It is now time to attempt to right the wrongs that may have existed so that others will not have to suffer the same.

In the early management and eventual resolution of any injustice, hurtful experience or loss, it is critical to look through the lens of a different perspective -- a viewpoint which sees the event as not one singular overwhelming attack, but more an event which is a part of a growth process. It requires a reshaping and purification process that will lead us over time to a better end and a higher plane of peacefulness - and dare I say, healing.

Steps for Coping with a Newly Acquired Hurt

1. **Recognize** it happened to you and whether it was intended or not. If it hurt or caused pain, damage control is needed. The hurt that you suffer today will build resilience and more strength as you manage it appropriately. As the Bible says, all things work to the good of those who love God and are called according to his purpose.

2. **Journalize** and write down in detail what you felt and experienced, and who witnessed the situation. It will be therapeutic to reduce the sting of the offense and will be useful if testimony regarding your issue is ever needed.

3. **Discuss** with your accountability partner(s) if you have one. If not, chose a wise person with whom you can speak in confidence. Depending upon the situation and with whom conflict occurs, consider privately informing your offender of what they did.

4. **Do not consider taking revenge** because to do so slows or prevents your healing rather than promoting it.

5. **Seek physical exercise** as soon as possible after the hurtful event and preferably with a friend. When you exercise, the body releases stress-reducing hormones.

6. **Do not hesitate to seek counseling...** People who have been disparaged and who have felt disrespected are highly sensitive to sharing, so they hide. Hiding means *'I can't let you know about this weakness or vulnerability because I already feel too bad. I just can't go there.'* So the tendency is to sweep things under the rug as if it will go away, but it doesn't. It festers. Keeping secrets or keeping it in darkness prolongs damage. When you verbalize it, you break it... calming it down, diffusing it and disintegrating its power. Spray light on it... spraying light on it promotes healing. In some cultures and traditions, it is considered shameful to reveal personal information. While I respect the culture, it's not a healthy choice.

7. **Resist believing you brought this upon yourself and/or possibly deserve what happened**. Pray for the ability to forgive no matter how ridiculous this process may seem.

"These troubles and sufferings of ours are, after all, quite small and won't last very long. Yet this short time of distress will result in God's richest blessing upon us forever and ever!"
- 2 Corinthians 4:17

My Seemingly Insurmountable Impairment

Initially my thoughts were, 'just quit.'

I finished all medical training in 1979. After 31 years, I became an Associate Dean of Students at St. Louis University School of Medicine. I served in that capacity from 2010-2018. My intention in service were altered dramatically when I began to lose my sight. Every aspect from my clinical practice to my ability to communicate with students was affected by this impending loss.

Vision Loss

My niece was getting married in 2013, and family was in town. That Saturday, I was waiting for my daughter and her husband to go up into the St. Louis Gateway Arch, instead of going up with them. All of a sudden, the vision in my right eye turned battleship grey -- 75% was grey, as if someone had painted it. Instead of telling them what had happened, I faked it and said, "I think I'm tired." I kept driving them around the town thinking if I lay down my vision will come back. My self-talk said, *Come on man, you're a doctor, what would you say if a patient told you I suddenly lost my vision?* Thinking that way didn't change my mind. I didn't tell anyone. Yes, my pride was in the way. I kept it to myself.

I had to walk her down the aisle the next day. I didn't want to ruin the day, so I kept it to myself.

I was seen on Monday and discovered I had a retinal detachment and needed emergency surgery.

Apparently, the condition was caused by my severe astigmatism - I had an oblong eyeball. Playing sports all my life, I'd been hit in the head and eye a few times, coupled with my severe myopia (near vision) contributed greatly.

The surgery stopped me from going blind completely in that eye. I was still able to function because my left eye was almost 20/20. Then glaucoma manifested in both eyes slowly over the years. They stopped me from driving in 2020, because my doctor said it was dangerous… "If my brother had the same vision as you, I would tell him don't drive. That's the same that I'm telling you."

I was angry… I was angry at God. *Lord, if you're in control and you have it all together, why would you let this happen to me? I need my vision to see patients and to do research! How is this going to work? How will I manage to serve without sight?*

I battled with God for nearly five years until I came to the resolution that God had His own plan.

In the meantime, frustration set in. I didn't hate Him, but I couldn't understand it. Then I began to comprehend when the Bible says, "Work out your salvation." What that means is each of us is on a private pathway with circumstances that we work with God to overcome. He will work it out, as long as we don't throw in the towel.

Gaining this understanding over time actually brought me into a deeper spiritual connection with God; one that I'd never had in my life. It was very difficult, yet it made me want to experience the living Words in the Bible - it being not just a document to recite, but a way to live.

I'm not just telling you what I haven't lived myself... The Bible says when you fall into diverse circumstances, through this situation, it will eventually lead to patience and completion. That takes work.

Dealing with Ghosts

The haunting involves having you stay the way you were as opposed to growing into the new place where God would have you be. I'm being haunted when I want to still feel sad, frustrated or angry about what happened to me instead of accepting the new path I have by overcoming the obstacles.

God allows adverse events because it serves His purpose - *Sometimes we have an answer as to why and sometimes we don't get one - but we still have to keep going.* I would have still been practicing medicine, teaching students, playing tennis and pursuing my own agenda, instead of asking God, *What do we do next?* - which is where we need to be - on His agenda, not ours.

So, though I still want to go fishing, I'm doing what I'm told; as a result of what happened, I felt an unction to share with you because God wants you to know that though bad things happen to Good people, he can use the challenges that you've had and are working through, to help other individuals, yourself and to serve His will.

About Hurt

Being hurt should not be a surprise, it should be expected. What God does not want us to do is continue to hurt - but continue to grow. You grow from your hurt.

How can one profit from suffering? Sometimes suffering is the profit. On the surface is the suffering (the physical and seen part), but how you manage it is the unseen part -- and that part is what works on the molding of your soul. The process of growth in terms of becoming more Christ-like - reaching total emotional, physical and spiritual health is about how we finish, not how we started. Growth demands us to experience and evolve.

Losing my vision and then experiencing hearing loss was a challenge I had to overcome to continue my purpose in Christ. And to fail at that, would have hindered my progress towards being all that Christ intended for me to be.

My pain and suffering has a point - so important that everyone shares in it. Nobody comes through life without experiencing it. It's God's modis operandi. We learn more from pain and suffering more than anything else in our lives, not the whole lot of fun we have.

I think about my bloody boot - I was walking along the side of a lake fishing and stepped on a spike. My boot filled with blood. As I pulled off my boot and allowed the blood to flow out, I decided then and there I would pay better attention and watch where I am stepping. It was a lesson I never forgot.

God teaches, trains and molds us through the suffering. Sometimes we play out God's will through our pain and suffering. As we respond to our pain and suffering in a way that is pleasing to God, we play out His will. Suffering gives us the ability to have perspective and the ability to make new choices.

Michael T. Railey, M.D.

My understanding of pain and suffering was enhanced, thus giving me the ability to share on a much deeper level than I would be able to achieve without the experiences. I've had a great many physical problems; I finally understood that I needed to be "prepared" and "qualified" to write this book and to teach how to see pain and suffering from God's perspective.

Addictions and Pornography

Filling the empty spaces is often what drives addictions.

Emotional eating is a battle for many of us. When we find ourselves in the middle of stuffing at 10:30 at night, stop and ask yourself, *"What do I really want right now that is causing me to eat this way?" If we're honest with ourselves, perhaps it's love, perhaps it's companionship, perhaps it's some type of confirmation?"*

Most of us never figure out what causes us to act this way and the habit takes over. We'll say, "That's just me," and give up. I don't think God wants us to stop. He wants us to figure it out. Let's work on it...

The truth is that the human body is remarkably constructed by God in such a way that almost anything we do repeatedly can lead to habituation - sometimes physiological, sometimes psychological. That cigarette, alcoholic beverage, extramarital sexual affair, shopping sales at the local department store, or the possession of a long coveted item can feel so satisfying that life without it seems not really worth living. **After a time, the body and mind do become dependent upon the experience of the immediate gratification and resists allowing us to stop re-experiencing.** It feels too good and the feelings of discomfort start if you try to stop.

These temporary pleasurable sensations for many people outweigh the danger that lie in their path. *When the mind and/or the body becomes accustomed to the sensation of pleasure, it sends out a message which encourages remaining in the behavioral pattern.*

This is the reason that bad habits are so hard to break... because they become a part of our everyday well-being, or so we think.

In reality, such a system as this can be used to our advantage rather than disadvantage. Especially if we could become accustomed to positive formative experiences instead of the deadly ones. The feelings we are seeking can be obtained in a safer and more consistent manner which is complimentary to longevity and healthy life as opposed to the self-suicide of bad habits. *It is our obligation and expected duty to not place in our bodies any substances which creates physiological or psychological addictions.* Romans 12:1-2 says it best; "I beseech you therefore brethren, by the mercies of God that ye present your bodies a living sacrifice, holy, acceptable unto God, which is your reasonable service."

It seems as if addictions towards everything is at an all-time high in America. People are eating, smoking, drinking, and snorting their way through life in a desperate manner as they seek temporary pleasure and rest from the stressors of daily living. In a country so bountifully blessed and full of potential for success, *What is behind this drive for immediate gratification in spite of consequences? What is that 'certain something' that we seek that would stop our self-destruction?*

Ms. Terry

My first visit with my patient Terry was notable, and set the tone for recognizing the source of her real problem.

"Doctor, it seems you expect me not to have anything fun in my life. If I don't drink and I don't smoke; I go to church and I don't fool around outside of my marriage, what pleasure is left for me? Doesn't everybody have something that they do?"

Terry's *health belief model* was a good example of what I call the "bingo" theory. Many people go through life feeling as if life is like a bingo game, in which each player/participant gets a free chip on the board to start the game. In their minds, that free chip is some physical or material entitlement which they have rationalized as needed and acceptable. A glass or two of wine before retiring... Maybe a cigarette at break time... A monthly secret session of intimacy with a co-worker... Justifying that this helps "tolerate" the marriage or make it through the circumstances of life.

Terry hears within her mind a tape from the past saying that if she is not experiencing continuous pleasure, life is not as full. With this life belief system in place, leading a disciplined life becomes an unpleasant and impossible duty. The selected habits we decide to justify might vary, but the message is the same.

...Since no one is perfect, pick your personal bad habit and stick with it. **This attitude prevents us from putting the effort into the painful process of change.** These entitlements can and do often become the crisis in our life which can eventually end our life. Living, believing that we each come equipped with a psychological cane to

lean on is faulty thinking. It leads to poor health outcomes secondary to the damages of the "vice" we have adopted. This tendency that exists today to seek out pleasure at all cost, is predicted in 2 Timothy 3:4. "This also know that in the last days perilous times shall come. For men shall be lovers of their own selves, covetous, boasters, proud, blasphemers, disobedient to parents, unthankful, unholy... Traitors, heady, highminded, lovers of pleasures more than lovers of God." The Biblical prediction is accurate as so many of us yield to the moment of our fleshly desires eventually later paying the price of physical and often family destruction.

Officer Kelly

Kelly is a police officer. He has a good job and a fine family. He states that he likes his job and is basically happy. Kelly can't stop smoking. His excuse is "I like my cigarettes." He is aware of all the risks associated with smoking, but feels that just three or four cigarettes a day is not that big of a deal. The ghost from his past is aware of the insecurities and anxieties which he has kept hidden and not dealt with since childhood. That voice of his subconscious rationalizes to him a favorite and effective line... *"Nobody is perfect. A few cigarettes a day relaxes me and is not nearly as bad the pack a day a lot of other people smoke."* **By thinking this way, his willingness to change is not triggered and his insecurities and anxieties are temporarily bathed in the physiologic effects of the drug nicotine.** In this particular case there was no discernable adverse childhood experience that was directly related to the smoking. It was more a case of sensing anxiety and fear during the course of the day and reacting by seeking the side effect provided by a smoke. The same calming effect might better be obtained by daily exercise, meditation and mindfulness techniques.

Making the substitution of a better habit for a lesser is not easy, but worthwhile to practice.

Al the Drinker

Al started drinking when he was in college with fraternity buddies. Almost everyone he associates with drinks to some extent. Consuming approximately four to six cans of beer most days of the week doesn't seem like much to him; especially since most of his buddies drink beer plus the "hard stuff" in the form of whiskey, vodka, or scotch. Since he feels pretty good, he is not impressed that his drinking is a problem. His personal ghost has convinced him of a lie. "If you were an alcoholic, you would feel drunk and be unable to function as well as you do. In your case drinking is just a fun and relaxing way of letting off steam, and no one is hurt."

Exchange Bad Habits for Healthy Addictions

There are many types of addictions. As earlier referenced, we can become addicted to just about anything; ranging from food to drugs to sex. There are also good (relatively) addictions. This includes exercising, socializing, laughter, art, writing, gardening, worship attendance, personal service, and music. The list of good things to do and become addicted to is lengthy. *Finding the balance among these selections in life is the key to a large portion of our success.* **When we develop the key to defeating one addiction, the same principles can be applied with some modifications to all. The solution to resisting any habit lies in starving the habit to death as we substitute another activity.** The voice of your "ghost" will become weaker and faint as the addiction becomes broken.

The key is to first develop a desire to change and then the persistence to substitute healthy behaviors for less healthy behaviors until the death of the habit is final. Spiritual support through personal prayer and prayer with friends and loved ones is mandatory as we tap into a strength which is beyond the natural. Most of us cannot develop this kind of courage without first eliminating some of the associated factors which weaken us to give in to habits. The great, late coach of the Green Bay Packers football team Vince Lombardi stated, "Fatigue makes cowards of us all." What does fatigue mean? This includes family problems, financial issues, physical fatigue, anger, frustration, relationship issues, unforgiveness and on and on. **When our emotions and strength is faded, our will to succeed is broken.**

To beat your addiction, you must first call out the issues (ghosts) that you do battle with which are often rooted in past experiences. Self-exploration, even if uncomfortable, may be necessary. It has been amazing to me the numbers of patients I've treated who started drinking alcohol or used some other substance because they were shy and needed "courage" to feel relaxed enough to cope with some social situations. The selected temporary bandage in these cases becomes the problem.

When resolution of those issues is recognized and dealt with, then the courage to deaden the addiction will emerge. It is vital to recognize what we wanted or needed to fill the "empty spaces" in our lives. The addictive substance in this case was just a filler to provide the sensation we thought we needed. **When the space is filled with the wrong thing, the problem will not go away, it is just covered up.** A shy person may be dealing with low self-esteem and certainly low confidence. When that need can either be diminished, eliminated, or coped with, we then stand at the gateway to victory. This kind of self-honesty often requires the help of a close friend or loved one to help us look at the truth of our various situations.

Addictions, although they may start unpredictably, continue in our lives and become soothing to us in order to fill a void or perceived need in our lives. Identification of the need and substitution with a more permanent healthier "balm" helps defeat the addiction at its source. Ultimately, heightened development of personal spirituality always contributes to the solution. We then must therefore do what it takes to get closer to and understand the word of God.

The Bible is loaded with wisdom in this area. The word of God provides us with a private counselor who keeps our confidence and doesn't charge us a penny. At the end of the next segment is a list which can be adapted to your situation to help cope with any addiction or habituation.

Pornography

Pornography is a very common addiction that especially affects men and Christians. At first glance, many would say pornography is a victimless crime, but it really isn't. It can become generational, can cause permanent emotional damage to the mate, it can warp sexual desire of the participant, it creates guilt, and can and does destroy marriages.

Due to its tremendous influence on families and the large industry that has developed in its wake, this addiction bears some separate and specific analysis in the next chapter. I am referring to pornography and the reading and viewing of sexually explicit materials. Entire books are often written on these addictions of various types. At this point, a touch of human physiology will be helpful. Within our brain is a rewards system. This system often is oversimplified to the term "dopamine system" In this particular area of the brain, positive feelings and emotions are rewarded by the release of a chemical called dopamine which rewards us with more positive sensation, but over time can leave us seeking a repeat performance. If the repeat experience is another mile walk in the park, the next day this is good. But, if the repeat action is to inhale or ingest a stimulant, this result is potentially damaging.

This system I have only touched upon is far more complicated than this introduction; however, it is not appropriate for great depth here. In addition to spiritual intervention, personal counseling, group therapy and the involvement of loving family members will also be required.

Frank and Jan - A Unique and Pervasive Addiction

It seemed as if everything was so complicated now between Frank and Jan in their seventh year of marriage. Even simple communications led to shouting matches. Eventually, they had separated, hoping that giving one another some space would rekindle their relationship. It was not working! Whenever they attempted to "patch things up," it was as if a wall would appear and they would be right back at each other with new arguments. Sex in the relationship was nonexistent. They were now into their sixth month with no intimacy between them.

Frank's job involved interacting with many women. He often found some co-workers attractive. One day a male friend called and convinced Frank to go along with him to a local adult club with exotic dancers performing. An inner voice (his ghost) seized the opportunity and spoke (again) to him, saying, "Everyone looks; and looking was certainly no sin."

Soon, on each Wednesday night, Frank and his buddy would drive over to the strip club to just have a good time and relax. They watched the women dance and would occasionally order drinks. Prior to this, Frank had fallen into the habit of looking at nude pictures of women in magazines and in X-rated movies. Many of his friends did this also, and Frank had convinced himself he was avoiding "actual sin" - and in some way was satisfying his ever increasing and frustrated sexual needs.

In actuality, this was false as looking at so much flesh only served to increase his yearning for sexual release and feed into him a warped sense of female sexuality. Each time Frank looked at Jan he became more disinterested and resentful of her. In some respect, he actually blamed her, in part, for his dilemma. Jan, even if she knew about it could never live up to the expectations and performance of an imaginary sexual relationship. This continued to make the relationship more tense. Frank began to edge closer to openly admiring other women and eventually sought out and found a sexual relationship outside of his marriage.

Sneaky Carl

Since childhood, Carl sneaked in his older brother's room to enjoy a secret stash of movies and magazines depicting sexual situations. The habit began when he was in the seventh grade. Often while visiting friends, they would all bring out photos and magazines and fantasize about having sex with the women they looked at. Now as an adult Carl subscribes to "girly" magazines explaining to his wife that this is normal behavior for men who really like sex. His wife does not understand this, but goes along with it. The voice of the ghost living in Carl's mind explained logically, "All men have sex drive, but some men have more than others. You have a very high sex drive and that's normal for you. I'll bet your hormone levels are higher than many other men." In reality, Carl was a very frustrated person. His life was not at all turning out as he would like. It was true that looking at the pictures and thinking sexual thoughts and masturbating gave him a temporary release from the world of confusion he felt he lived in.

In truth, Carl's heightened libido was more related to multiple personal issues including personal low self-esteem, and a need for affirmation as a desirable person. This was complicated by his financial, and vocational stresses. Sex served as self-medication to soothe temporarily some of his anxiety and tension. He thought he longed for women like those in the magazines, but deep down inside he longed for control over his life along with attention and validation as a person and as a man.

His relationship with his wife was always troubled. Their blunted sexuality was only a symptom of much more deeply rooted problems between the two of them. The women he fantasized about performed to his specifications and offered no resistance. The more he looked, the more he lusted. These persistent thoughts eventually led Carl to act out sexually in an attempt to now satisfy the great need which he believes has welled up inside of him demanding satisfaction. The real issue of resolving the conflict between he and his mate was lost in the smokescreen of confusion and personal dishonesty he lived with.

The Fallout

It feels so good to satisfy the sensation of what we feel we want; and seems so natural when we get what we think we need. Sex, what was originally intended as a gift for our marriage; accentuating a bond of intimacy and providing a means of procreation has been warped. In a marriage, the conflict over differing sexual drives can become a point of contention.

Pornography is a most effective tool for the **enemy** of God in impeding the development of normal healthy sexual appetites and relationships, thus increasing the possibilities of broken marriages and families in the wake of the problem -- thereby sidetracking us from obtaining true Godly sexual intimacy between mates, which was the original intent. The pornographic problem is generally more common among men, as the male of our specie has always been most susceptible to visual sexual imagery by God's design. In America, more money is spent on pornography than on bread consumption.

Sex, Sex, Sex

With the creation of man and woman was the "eye gate," stimulating the male to seek a mate and reproduce after his own kind, which was critical to the populating of humanity.

Unfortunately, in our modern society there has been a tremendous perverting of the natural sexual drives of men and women. The type of intimacy we are encouraged to seek now goes far beyond the confines of physical sex in marriage only. Too many want to substitute sex as a universal balm for all problems, wanting sex to ease the pain in our lives like ointment to an open wound.

Have Frustrations and Woes? Just Have Sex! NO! The problem is that the gratification we get is temporary, uncommitted, shallow, and psychologically damaging. Further, pornography conveys unrealistic expectations to and for our real life partner; and sets a standard totally outside of the relationship. Unfair comparisons are created - which our mates must now unknowingly live up to. Pornographic material is not just the hard core "X-rated" type of visual experience, but there are also many other lesser variations extending from lingerie ads to "soft porn" as demonstrated in movies, soap operas, and on various television programs. These forms of pornography can be just as addictive and damaging.

Many argue that sexual drive and sexuality is normal, and justify all forms of its expression based on the nature. Thinking that a 'natural drive' compels us to act. We question why we were we given this if not to use it; and blaming God for providing us with such a powerful temptation to do battle with constantly.

However, we should not blame God for the natural, unnatural tendencies and perversions we want to fulfill through intercourse. True, these drives are given and allowed by God, but are placed for a specific purpose. Procreation is the first necessary reason, and the gift of shared pleasurable intimacy to promote and maintain bonding of married couples is another. The original plan was one of order, pleasure, and shared intimacy for us and not domination over us. God does not give us sex and then snatch it back.

The world now views sex as recreational; like a game of tennis or racquetball as we change from partner to partner. Because of the physiological relaxation which occurs after sex, many now use God's gift as a therapy technique to sooth away daily anxieties and tensions, thus converting lovemaking into an addictive process for relief. This opiate, as it is with all addictive habits and substances carries a number of side effects including psychological trauma, unwanted pregnancy, disease, and even death.

Unfortunately, the consequences of our sexual immoralities have delayed effects as we move from person to person thinking that since we feel no immediate consequences, everything must be fine. We are told to flee fornication and that we are sinning against our body in and that whatsoever we sow, we reap. (1 Corinthians 6:18 and Galatians 6:7-8) However, the consequences do collect and can manifest themselves so far down the line that we lose sight of where the origin of the problem started.

Pete the Player

Pete spent the majority of his youth in multiple casual sexual relationships over many years. His attitude and opinion of women became so poor that he eventually found he trusted no woman. He had affairs with married women, with his friends, ex-girlfriends, and even with co-workers. The memory of sexual situations and liaisons he had accumulated eventually warped him to the point that he was unsuitable for a good relationship with anyone. Through deeper conversation, *Pete admitted he was preoccupied with porn at a young age, which likely contributed to his life path.*

Once the pornographic spirit takes root, it is virtually impossible to not see the opposite sex as an object for satisfaction of desires instead of a person. When the seeds of addiction are initiated, the haunting of our thoughts to continue the addictive behavior will continue if you let it, on to your eventual ruin.

We are warned Biblically that the sins of the father are visited upon the sons and for many generations thereafter in Exodus. I have not seen men who lived lives of casual intimate contacts escape from life without a backlash of their deeds having a devastating effect both on themselves, family members and their children. Once sexual immorality develops a stronghold, family destruction and generational repetition is not far behind. Disturbing normal relationships is satan's goal. **Now that you know that, you can make choices to free yourself of those strongholds.**

A Plan for Defeating the Strongholds of (Addictions and) Pornography

Pornography comes in many forms. Addiction to sex and pornography is quite common. When you find yourself stimulated, be on the alert. In America, more money is spent each year on pornography than dollars spent on bread. When children are subjected to adult materials, the seeds for a dangerous addiction are planted as well. Once established these addictions have an effect on our relationships and can ruin marriages and families. Every effort must be made to avoid exposure to sexually explicit materials in order to starve this addiction and regain control. Review the steps below several times to help your subconscious mind obtain a firm grasp on what to do when challenges arise. This is a problem worth the effort to defeat.

1. It is critical that we first recognize pornographic addictions as a problem! The natural man or woman within wants to seek out fleshly relief. When you yield to those desires, you feed them and their growth will become uncontrollable. Romans 7:23-24 states, "But I see another law at work in me, waging war against the law of my mind

and making me a prisoner of the law of sin at work within me. What a wretched man I am! Who will rescue me from this body that is subject to death? I can sense Paul (the writer's), great difficulty as he obviously has had some experience with the frustration of trying to overcome fleshly and even sexual weaknesses. But the battle is on, and success is in sight once you establish you have a problem!

2. Find an accountability partner who will agree to demand honesty on your part and hold your feet to the fire of sexual morality. We need earthly help through our associations in obtaining and maintaining sexual morality. The Bible teaches that "As iron sharpens iron, so one person sharpens another," Proverbs 27:17. It is wise to make preset agreements with a godly friend who you must be accountable to on trips and any situations where sexual immorality can occur.

3. Restrict illicit sexual images and sounds by reducing television, magazine, social media and internet visual and auditory stimulus. Exposing yourself to that which you know feeds into the stimulation of your senses is asking for trouble. Others may not understand that for you a program with heavy sex scenes and nudity is like parading cocaine in front of an addict. If you keep watching, you will eventually become a participant. Our instruction from the word of God is clear. "For all that is in the world, the lust of the flesh, and the lust of the eyes, and the pride of life is not of the father, but is of the world." 1John 2:16

4. Flee sexual situations (with people an images), without justification or rationalization. The word flee is not a soft word, as it means to actively and in a straightforward manner run away from situations which could lead to sexual involvement. Everything starts with a thought. When you think it, avoid it or replace it. You cannot win a debate with the devil; as your eyes will betray your good intentions. Just run. Removing yourself from a situation is often the only thing you can do before it is too late.

5.   Ask God for forgiveness of past sexual indiscretions. He will be willing to forgive you. (Ephesians 5:4) This clears the slate with God if you are sincere, thus removing guilt, establishing and giving you a new opportunity to gain victory!

6.   Fight to discover, and then resolve emotional issues which could lead to a need for excessive quenching of your sexual thirst. The "balm" of sexuality is frequently a choice to replace another need that we might have (Examples: loneliness, relationship hunger, anxiety and fear, low self-esteem, and anger release.) Go after what you really need, instead of the substitute of a "sexual band aid."

7.   *What are you supposed to do?* Find a suitable husband or wife. Burning with passion is not healthy, and thus complicates being single. If you do not have the gift of celibacy (which most of us don't) you must use your sexual drive as a motivator to begin the process of seeking a mate in earnest and marry. Intimacy in marriage provides us with the correct avenue of expression for our sexual needs as God planned. The marital bed is undefiled (Hebrews 13:4) and we should drink deeply from our own well! By Biblical instruction, enjoy sex with your mate forsaking lusting after others. At times physical or emotional challenges complicate our intimacy. Discuss and do your best to fix and resume normal sexual activities.

Otherwise, marital problems often become greater. Good communication between partners is the foreplay that leads to satisfying sexual relationships.

8. Pray daily (1Thes. 5:17) to increase your spiritual growth and to remain connected to your source of strength. This requires discipline. Ask God to give you the discipline you need and then help yourself by setting aside a time of day which you jealously protect. *(The forces of evil will do anything to take away from your time, focus and consistency, which is why you need to schedule and keep your schedule no matter what.)*

9. Never be shamed into giving up. Failure or temporary setbacks can happen. Press on to the result you are seeking.

10. I suggest that each spouse join a ministry or group to gain support from other couples, individually or together. Your mate can play a vital role in helping you overcome problems. This is another reason why knowing your mate well and having a personal friendship is important before marriage. Marital partners who don't have good pre-marital relationships generally experience trouble in the marital bed at some time. The main cause is usually again communication problems.

11. Fasting, coupled with prayer can intensify your progress to obtain the result you need. Fasting allows us to connect and to gain God's answers, mercy and grace because it allows us to eliminate distractions that often keep us disconnected. When we successfully deprive ourselves of fleshly desires, we gain spiritual insight, willpower and focus through fasting.

Patterns, Generational Curses, and Family Spirits

This is a topic that makes us a little nervous at first mention. I think the primary reason is because it has not been taught to us, and most of us don't understand it. So, let us begin slowly and simply with a few facts. Unfortunately, your good looks and charming ways are not the only things passed on to you from your ancestors.

We must also consider characteristics we have that are not so pleasant could also be derived from a grandparent, parent or a distant uncle or aunt. Sometimes that tendency to gamble or drink whiskey, commit crimes, or chase the opposite sex is shared by many in the family and/or is inherited.

A book that deals with problems and challenges from our past would be incomplete without considering possibilities of familiar patterns, habits, and potentially curses. Let us begin with what I believe to be the simplest of these terms, best described as patterns and pathways.

A few years ago our mailman exhibited an odd change in his delivery pattern. To save time and effort, he began to walk across my yard instead of using the stairs and driveway. We did not notice this until the grass began to die in his path from use. Apparently, other service persons noticed the path and began to use it as well. Over time, we developed a bare brown dirt path through our lawn. This was quite disturbing, and an action plan was needed.

As referenced often in *Living with a Ghost*, there is power in recognition. Recognition can often, if we let it, throw open the doors to recovery and successful management. As you scan your family tree, is there evidence of patterns and habits that are similar to yours? Most of us would agree, there is, if we are honest. Patterns of teen pregnancy, alcoholism, drug abuse, obesity and/or certain diseases are patterns in families.

Patterns and habits are not always bad; they can be good,,, for example, a family which has developed a legacy of attending and graduating from a certain school. A pattern in our family was reading; our parents would read to us as children and would often give us books as gifts. As siblings, we would at times read to each other, and our children and grandchildren have followed suit.

These paths and habits, if unchecked can become like a generational curse, which is invoked not by spoken words or incantations, but from actual repetitive behaviors.

In my family, I have counted among my five brothers and sisters and their children a total of 16 divorces. No one in the family has ever brought this to us to share and discuss. I have thought how interesting it would be if a few divorced and remarried or even not remarried, commented on what they discerned over time was the root cause of the problem. Maybe it hints of how they would rewrite the narrative if they could. This could be a profitable family experience if recognition of repetitive trends were seen and a few people decided to construct an action plan.

One of the famous series of similar behavior traits is given to us in the, Bible, Genesis 20:26 where we learn the story of Abram lying about Sarah being his sister and not his wife to protect his own life. A few chapters later, Abraham's son Isaac gets into a situation where he feels the need to lie that Rebecca, his wife, is instead, his sister. Then, just like a chip off the block, Esau lies to Issac about his identity to trick his brother's birthright to himself.

Clearly patterns, followed by development of pathways, and habits can be dangerous. Unfortunately, some bad habits tend to team up with others that match well, such as cigarettes and alcohol or lying and cheating.

There is great power in recognition, and even greater power in a willingness to change. Let us recall some of our past discussions. Before sincere change can be enacted, there must first be recognition and the beginnings of a commitment to "I don't want to be that person anymore" or "I don't want to continue this habit anymore!"

Let's recall my analogy about mailpersons wearing out a spot in my lawn until it became a path. I did not recognize it until it began to take on a new appearance, and also not until others had joined in the destruction. I have heard it expressed like this: Spirits have a gang mentality. As they experience success, they invite like-minded spirits to join them, making the chances to stop them more difficult.

You initially may be overeating out of frustration and a need to self-medicate. This spirit is soon joined by spirits of overindulgence and banqueting, followed soon by reveling and self-comfort through alcohol or smoking. The gang is complete when "discouragement" joins. You have now acquired a personal band of spiritual thugs to do battle. So, the sooner you come to recognition and "Fight! Fight! Fight!" the better off you will be.

A next logical question should be, "Where do these spirits come from and how do we acquire these familiar general trouble makers and demons?"

Spirits and Demons

This is a topic which we must not allow to frighten us as it is real and can and should be managed.

There are many theories on the sources of these entities.

The God we serve is good and requires obedience. His opposing enemy and therefore our enemy as well is evil. It is manifested in the character of satan as adversary and the fallen angels, spirits, and/or demons he directs in his personal war against us as the children of God.

Regardless of the original source of the addiction - an ancestral tie or a new tie, the management/first step is the same. The behavior has to be eliminated in the present. In other words, if one got drinking from grandpa and daddy, or if he got it from partying with a group of friends, the behavior needs to be interrupted and stopped now, in the present, and then replaced with a different pattern or habit.

The spirit is waiting to be invited in - the spirit of over indulgence and intemperance... a drink once or twice a week isn't enough... I need a beer every morning, and have opened a door and welcomed the spirits of reveling and overindulgence.

I like beer, and my father liked beer, and the rumor was that my dad's biological father liked beer, though he was adopted. So, I don't drink very often to avoid inviting the spirit in.

Watch out! I never saw my father "drunk" because he likely did it constantly at a low level and his body got accustomed to it - allowing the spirit to flourish and get stronger. For all I know, addictions breed liars, and liars hide habits.

Alcoholics often hide their bottles... *How can you tell if an alcoholic or drug addict is lying? "If his mouth is moving!"* It may seem harsh, but it's true. That spirit invites the lying and the lying supports the habit and keeps the portal open. In any addiction, lying is a significant symptom - because the addicted person has to always protect their addiction.

These spirits desire a place to live, reside and influence. When we fall into negative influences which are against God's Word or unknowingly invite these spirits to take up residency, then we are hooked. Often in our families, we demonstrate by our behaviors, thoughts, actions and lifestyle which directly impact the development of what we later refer to as a generational or familiar curse. Although the depth and breadth of the problems certainly vary from one family to the next, the general plan of satan still works until we recognize these attacks and strive to defeat them!

Our God will always provide us with a way out of every trap satan lays for us.

Steps to Activating Spirit

1. **Recognition** - Spend some time alone on more than one occasion taking note of familiar traits, illnesses, and events both good and bad. You must be willing to admit that a change needs to be made, recognizing that all that feels good to you is not good for you. Once you make the connections to the undesired and negative issues, decide to address them and choose to remain continuously dedicated and committed to their/its elimination.

2. **Confirmation** - Consider speaking with other family members or loved ones after prayer to obtain their thoughts. Praying prior to your conversation will support your choice and desire to eliminate the undesirable and negative problem. It's also important to pray because you'll need discernment to determine who to ask, as you don't want to ask the wrong person for good advice because they will give poor or inadequate advice.

"Blessed is the man that walketh not in the counsel of the ungodly, nor standeth in the way of sinners, nor sitteth in the seat of the scornful." - Psalm 1:1

Yes, you love your buddy, your partner or loved one, but they may not be willing or capable of taking this new pathway with you. The purpose of choosing a loved one or relative to have a conversation with is to confirm and perhaps offer insight into the past and/or the problem you sense you are experiencing.

3. **Action Planning** - Now that you've identified the concerns and problems, choose a plan of action which you can commit to in mind, body, spirit and habit that will

begin to lead to successful change. This includes, writing, thinking, acting and eliminating any undesired tendencies which would interrupt your progress.

4.   **Sustaining Change** - Don't be alarmed if you encounter resistance, both internal and external. The people who are accustomed to you as you are (were) will not want you to change. Drinking buddies and eating buddies always want you to keep drinking and eating with them.

5.   **Focus on Consistency** - Internal change requires your unwavering commitment, and it will be difficult. Working on you should be your focus. Memorizing and reciting scripture is your offensive weapon - it's the only way to fight back against the negative forces of evil which seek to keep you the same. As you pray, focus on scripture and experience new outcomes, you will begin to feel different. This is the prime time to "Put on the whole amour of God," because the battle is at its greatest intensity at this time. Evil knows you want to eliminate it.

6.   **Revealing Leads to Complete Healing** - Always consider root causes as you seek answers reconsidering adverse childhood experiences if applicable. People want to sweep root causes under the rug because they are so nasty. If Uncle Tony took you to "tickle time" in the basement, the natural tendency would be to try and forget it. The way to heal is to talk about it, name it - YES, he abused me, OR YES, I got jumped during the summer when I was 13 years old and nobody saved me. I was bullied. It messed me up and I'm ashamed, hurt, scared and angry... so I cannot resist looking over my shoulder.

When we ignore what happened, we will never recover from it. We MUST be willing to look at the root and then kill it... You've got to deal with what happened to you.

7. **Counseling Matters** - Do not hesitate to seek counseling at any time. Sharing with a trusted professional will allow you to unburden areas you may have avoided or kept secret. As you release in conversations, you invite healing. A key to healing is forgiveness - forgiving yourself is difficult, yet essential to the process.

8. **Fellowshipping Matters** - Seek out and maintain fellowship with a church of choice. Keeping in mind that your personal road is between you and God, primarily. The relationship with the church is an aide. Being connected with fellow believers encourages the relational connections that Christ supports in healing and forgiveness.

9. **Stay positive during battle.** Speak positively to yourself and reward yourself for successes by keeping a personal journal of progress. Seeing what you've changed and how you've handled issues along the way will encourage you when you face challenges. Also, taking your successes to a friend/support group will provide you with external success confirmation.

10. **Express gratitude out loud.**
Maintaining gratefulness at all times for your blessings is a must. Doing so, you will notice your resilience in life is enhanced.

11. **Memorize and then recite scripture daily**. You must memorize scripture that applies to the problems you seek to improve.

It destroys the strongholds of generational curses. Every phrase or sentence of memorized scripture brings you a little closer to thinking like the Word of God.

"Finally, brethren, whatsoever things are true, whatsoever things are honest, whatsoever things are just, whatsoever things are pure, whatsoever things are lovely, whatsoever things are of good report; if there be any virtue, and if there be any praise, think on these things."
- Philippians 4:8

Late Night Snacks
(Insert Drinking, Drugs, Shopping)

If your habit is eating late night snacks filled with sugar and or salt, it may be a food addiction tied to emotional eating. You know it's bad for your health and yet you continue to do it. *What's the solution?*

First, be honest with yourself and figure out what you really want - *What are you substituting this food for?* Answer that honestly.

a) Is it really intimate conversation with a mate or friend that you're not able to get, and that's why you're eating?
b) Is it an expression of affection that you really want right now, and that's why you eat?
c) Is there something that happened to you that you really want to discuss, but you've not shared or expressed it?

These are all common realities that we try to substitute food (or drugs, alcohol) for. Do you have an answer? Likely you do. Grab a notebook and write what you are feeling and thinking. This will assist you in processing what's been happening. It won't be easy; however, it's a start to breaking the cycle.

Those kind of emotional substitutions are never satisfying. Ultimately, they may fill up your stomach or mind and give you a false sense of fulfillment - but they don't really satisfy completely, your need. (So, if you need a hug, sex, intimacy, companionship, or simply to vent, and that hasn't happened, you'll still have the need in the morning).

Changing your mind and the habit itself is what will free you to eliminate what's not working and draw near what you need to experience fulfilment.

Make the Decision to Break the Habit

The plan should be at least three fold:

1. Substituting the carbs for protein for a period of time.
2. Writing in your journal what you're doing, how you're feeling and what you intend to do.
3. Exploring the other areas that you are lacking as you read, memorize and repeat scripture out loud during repeated intervals.

Yes, it's work. Dedication and perseverance over this will lead to success over many areas. **What you have just done is created a new biological microchip for your mind to take a new path leading to a different outcome.**

Take this example and apply it to gambling, pornography or heart disease as a generational issue. When you've been exposed to these things in your past, either witnessing or being born into certain conditions, they often have long term effects on your decision making and activities. You must make a conscious choice to first recognize and then rid the impact (issue) from your life.

Colossians 3 tells us to set our affection on things above not on earth and, specifies us to: **Mortify** therefore thy deeds which are on earth such fornication, uncleanness, evil planning, and covetousness which is idolatry.

What does this mean? You must deaden pathways and portals in your life that are leading to self-destructive behaviors.

Change to an activity which could disrupt your improper thoughts, as soon as your recognize what is happening. Think about and repeat a scripture out loud multiple times. Take a walk. Or get up, go to another room, and return a phone call if necessary. The key is to change your thoughts. You must remember, as you think, you become -- you have to constantly monitor your thought patterns and redirect them into correct pathways.

These actions which again alter your thinking, your habits and your environment can be lifesaving as you build a new path in your mind bypassing the old ways keeping you hostage to the world's (substance abuse)/internet's (pornography) dark side.

Over time, you will feel a burst of reward like sensation as your resistance increases in power.

Finally, report your recent success to your accountability partner to gain more sense of reward, success, and personal self-control.

I know this is not easy. The battle you fight each day could be sourced in ancestors naturally you never met. People who are in your family line could have developed habits or gene sequences that came out of circumstances you know nothing about, and they were passed onto you. We don't have any control over the patterns or habits that come from our ancestors, but we can control and alter those which we have inherited.

For example, I can do nothing about my grandfather's gambling, but I can do something about not gambling myself.

My dad's biological father is unknown to me and to him. We don't know what habits he brought into our line, but we know what we don't want to do.
If diabetes runs in your family line, make choices to avoid becoming pre-diabetic with diet, exercise and attitude.

We have no understanding or explanation of the behaviors of the people who came before us, but we certainly have the right to block the effects of those negative influences on our personal lives. In fact, we have an obligation to break free from the effects of those influences.

Be a curse breaker.

Take pride in knowing that your efforts are helping to eradicate a familiar and familial spirit which live on in power if you do not continue your heroic fight.

Getting personal counseling and or group therapy may be helpful. I applaud all efforts to fight against these familiar spirits.

Attempts for self-improvement are not to obtain perfection. What we are working to do is to reduce dysfunctional and damaging behaviors.

Additionally, expect occasional setbacks or failure. Being too hard on ourselves is what our enemy wants. No truly successful individual would tell you that they never had a setback. Comebacks are part of all successful journeys.

Dr. Railey's Adapted Words of Encouragement

Memorizing and utilizing words of wisdom and encouragement based on Scripture can be your help in times of need.

- God is your strength. Learn to rely on His power and might.

- The enemy is unable to stand against God's might.

- Evil surrounds us whether we see it or not. Do not be deceived.

- Arm yourself to stand, shielded and protected by the Lord.

- Be truthful, do not lie. Make honorable choices.

- Don't run to trouble. Walk toward peaceful outcomes.

- Standing in faith allows you to deflect triggers which used to draw you in to old behaviors. Faith is your shield as you know that you don't have to resort to past behaviors because you are renewed in your mind. (The Mind of Christ)

- Scripture is your offensive weapon - protecting your mind and thoughts, freeing you from your past, offering a new future. The presence of the Holy Spirit leads to your new destiny through activating the Word of God whenever negative or evil thoughts or words spoken try to fight you. The Word is your sword.

- Every single day pray and stay connected to God no matter what.

This wisdom is based on my interpretation of Ephesians 6:10-18...
I adapted these words from scripture with the intent of showing you that you can implant them into your heart, mind and life so that when you get into certain situations, they will come alive, becoming the agent you need to solve your problems and change your situation.

Scriptural Glossary

My Thinking

- As a man (or woman) thinks, so he is... Proverbs 23:7

- Finally my brethren; whatsoever thoughts are true, whatsoever thoughts are honest, whatsoever thoughts are just, whatsoever thoughts are pure, whatsoever thoughts are lovely, whatsoever thoughts are of good report, if there be any virtue or praise, then think on these things... Philippians 4:8

- Take captive every thought and bring it into obedience with Christ. 2 Corinthians 10:5

Worry and Anxiety

- Do not be anxious about anything. Philippians 4:6

- Cast all your cares on Him. 1 Peter 5:7

- He who has begun a good work in you will complete it. Philippians 1:6

Overindulgences and Addictions

- Know ye not that your body is a temple... 1 Corinthians 6:19

- And every man that striveth for the mastery is temperate in all things... 1 Corinthians 9:25

Suffering

- Count it all joy when ye fall into diverse temptations. James 1:2

- And the God of all grace, who called you to his eternal glory in Christ, after you have suffered a little while, will himself restore you and make you strong, firm and steadfast. 1 Peter 5:10

- For our light and momentary troubles are achieving for us an eternal glory that far outweighs them all. 2 Corinthians 4:17

Acknowledgments

Thank you to my wife Mary - without whose love and support, this could never have been completed. I love and cherish you.

To my children Shaliss, Kenyon, and Charis - it is my prayer that this book be inspirational to you.

To my father Raymond Stephen Railey, who taught me responsibility, character and the importance of honesty.

To Tyree Edward Miller and Jessica Ouyang, MD discussions with you about real life cases has been invaluable. Thank you both.

Kappa Alpha Psi Fraternity, Incorporated. Thank you for helping me become the man that I am.

To my patients over the years who trusted me with their health management and taught me by their challenges and victories.

Saint Louis University School of Medicine; I appreciate the opportunity to have seen my patients through a spiritually based institution.

Thank you to Pastor Miki Merritt of New Cote Brilliante Church of God - God bless you for your guidance and leadership. And much appreciation to the Men of Issachar - our discussions and Bible Study have been invaluable.

Thank you to my writing coach and publisher Jo Lena Johnson. Thank you for your coaching, expertise and professionalism.

About the Author

Michael T. Railey, MD, is a graduate of the St. Louis College of Pharmacy, University of Missouri School of Medicine, and the University of Florida Family Medicine Residency training program. He is Professor Emeritus Community and Family Medicine, retired and past Associate Dean Diversity, Equity, Inclusion from 2010 to 2017, at Saint Louis University. He currently serves as student advisor and consultant to Vice Dean of Department of Diversity, Equity, and Inclusion. Dr. Railey assists in maintaining pre-existing programs from recruitment, and retention, to pipeline and development programming. He is a member of Alpha Omega Alpha Medical Honor Society and also, Kappa Alpha Psi Fraternity, Incorporated.

Dr. Railey was the first Family Medicine Clerkship Director at Saint Louis University and has also been Chief Medical Officer for St. Louis County. He has written book chapters, magazine articles, and journal publications in the areas of obesity, spirituality and medical care, stress management without drugs, and health disparities in the St. Louis, Missouri, area. He remains committed to community service and has been involved in collaborations with the American Health Association, and the Mound City Medical Forum. Dr. Railey is now semi-retired and enjoying life with his wife Mary Paulette; they are the parents of three adult children and have three grandchildren.

www.ingramcontent.com/pod-product-compliance
Lightning Source LLC
Chambersburg PA
CBHW042321090526
44585CB00024BA/2739